JO GRAY

Ageless Beauty with Oats: Secrets to Hydrating Your 40+ Skin

Contents

One

Understanding Dry Skin in Mature Ages

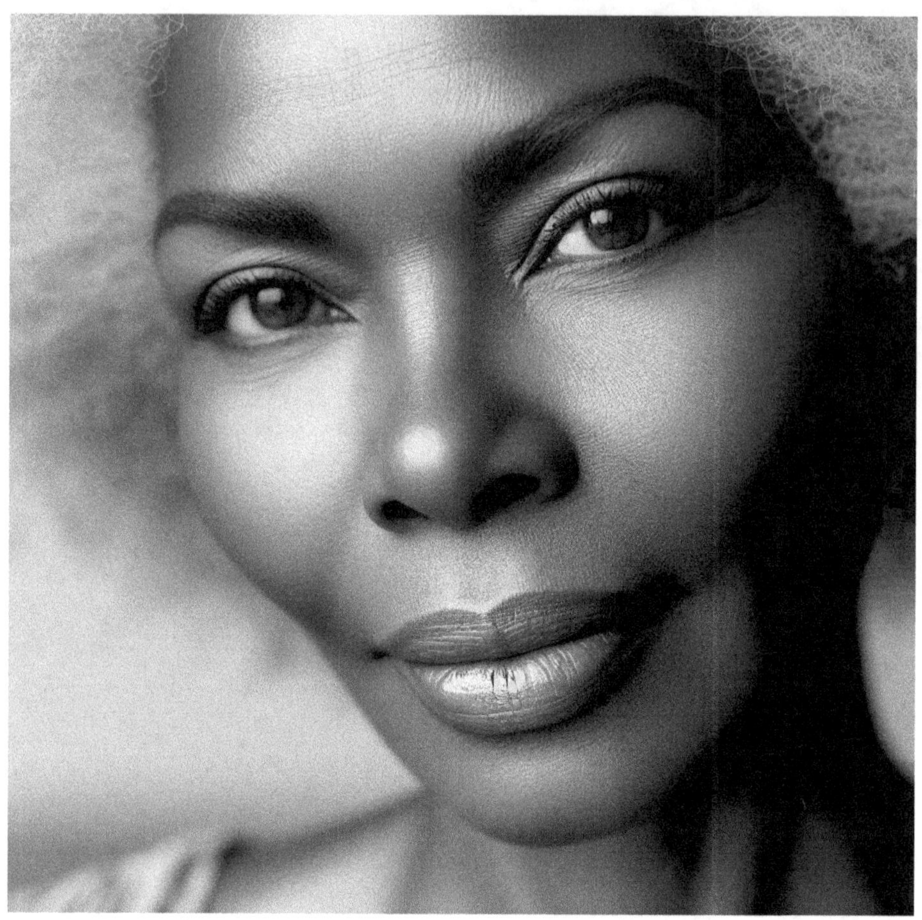

Ah, the dew-kissed glow of youth. We remember it fondly, that time when skin bounced back with a youthful resilience, seemingly impervious to the passage of time. But as the years gracefully pass, our skin whispers a different story. It becomes drier, thinner, etched with the wisdom of experience, and perhaps a little more prone to the whispers of dryness.This is not a cruel twist of fate, but a natural chapter in our skin's ever-evolving narrative. Like loyal friends, collagen and elastin, the proteins that once kept our skin plump and bouncy, begin a gentle retreat. Hyaluronic acid, the moisture-magnet that holds onto water like a thirsty camel, slowly starts saying its goodbyes. And hormonal shifts, like the quiet waltz of menopause, further disrupt the delicate dance of skin hydration and oil production.

The world outside, too, plays its part. Sun exposure, our old nemesis, leaves behind a legacy of dryness and wrinkles. Pollution, the unwelcome guest in our urban jungles, further stresses our skin's defenses. And let's not forget the harsh whisper of central heating, sucking the moisture from the air like a thirsty dragon.

But fear not, dear reader! This is not a one-way street. While dry skin in our mature years presents unique challenges, it also opens the door to fascinating discoveries. We get to explore the intricate world of skin science, where humectants, emollients, and occlusives (moisturizing ingredients that prevent water loss) become our new friends, working in concert to keep our skin hydrated and happy.

And in this exploration, we'll encounter a surprising hero: oatmeal. Not the breakfast staple you know, but a finely milled, colloidal form that unlocks a treasure trove of skin-loving benefits. Its gentle touch soothes irritation, its humectant properties draw in moisture, and its anti-inflammatory powers calm the whispers of dryness.

So, join us on this journey, dear reader, as we delve into the fascinating world of mature skin. We'll uncover the science behind dryness, explore the natural wonders of hydration, and discover the humble oatmeal's surprising role in keeping our skin radiant, resilient, and eternally beautiful, in every chapter of our lives.

Resources for further exploration:

- American Academy of Dermatology: https://www.aad.org/public/every day-care/skin-care-secrets/anti-aging/maximize-anti-aging-products
- Mayo Clinic: https://www.mayoclinichealthsystem.org/hometown-he alth/speaking-of-health/what-to-do-about-dry-skin

This is just the beginning, dear reader. In the next section, where we'll delve deeper into the specific challenges of dry skin 40+ and discover the magic of oatmeal in action!

Two

The Magic of Oatmeal for Ageless Beauty

Oatmeal – the warm, comforting breakfast staple that fueled warriors and poets alike – holds a surprising secret: it's nature's ageless beauty secret. For centuries, cultures around the world have lauded its skin-loving properties, using it in baths, poultices, and even facial masks.

But what makes this humble grain so potent? Let's crack open the treasure chest of oats and unveil its hidden gems:

Oatmeal: Nature's Hydrating Heroine

Forget diamonds; oats are a girl's (and boy's!) best friend. Packed with nutrients like B vitamins, vitamin E, zinc, and magnesium, oats nourish the skin from within. And just like a sponge soaks up water, oats excel at attracting and retaining moisture, thanks to their high starch and beta-glucan content. These natural humectants act like tiny magnets, drawing water to your skin and keeping it plump and hydrated.

But oats don't stop there. Colloidal oatmeal, a finely milled form, takes hydration to a whole new level. Its ultra-fine particles gently exfoliate dead skin cells, revealing a brighter, smoother complexion, while its anti-inflammatory properties soothe irritation and calm redness – a common foe of dry, mature skin.

Unlocking the Anti-Aging Power of Oats

Think of oats as time travelers, journeying back to your youthful skin. They stimulate the production of collagen and elastin, the magic duo that keeps our skin bouncy and wrinkle-free. This isn't just wishful thinking; scientific studies have shown that colloidal oatmeal can increase collagen synthesis by up to 50%!

Not only do oats fight wrinkles, but they also act as nature's shield against environmental aggressors. Their antioxidant power helps combat free radical damage, the main culprit behind premature aging. So, the next time you step out into the sun, remember, oats have your back (and your face!).

Tailoring Your Oatmeal Regimen: A DIY Symphony for Your Skin

Just like snowflakes, no two skins are alike. So, to unlock the full potential of your oat-powered beauty routine, listen to your skin's unique whispers. Are you battling dryness? Honey, yogurt, avocado, and aloe vera will join your oat party, infusing your mask with an extra dose of moisture.

Wrinkles giving you the side-eye? Vitamin C, retinol, and alpha-hydroxy acids (AHAs) are your wrinkle-fighting allies. Team them up with oats, and watch your fine lines fade into oblivion.

Hyperpigmentation got you down? Licorice root, niacinamide, and kojic acid will be your melanin-busting buddies. Mix them with oats, and get ready to embrace a brighter, more even skin tone.

And for those fighting the good fight against gravity, peptides, green tea extract, and squalane are your firming forces. Add them to your oat mask, and let your skin defy the pull of time.

Remember, the beauty of DIY masks is their endless possibilities. Don't be afraid to experiment with seasonal ingredients like pumpkin puree in autumn or cucumber slices in summer. The key is to listen to your skin and let your creativity blossom.

So, dear reader, ditch the expensive creams and embrace the magic of oatmeal. With a little DIY spirit and a dash of nature's goodness, you can unlock the ageless beauty that lies within. Remember, you are the artist, and your skin is your canvas. Let's paint a masterpiece, one oat-infused brush stroke at a time.

Ready to get started? Here are some simple oat mask recipes to inspire you:

The Hydrating Hero:

- 1/4 cup ground oatmeal
- 2 tablespoons plain yogurt
- 1 tablespoon honey

Mix all ingredients into a smooth paste. Apply to clean, dry skin and leave on for 15-20 minutes. Rinse with warm water and pat dry.

The Wrinkle Warrior:

- 1/4 cup ground oatmeal
- 1 teaspoon vitamin C serum
- 1/2 teaspoon avocado oil

Combine all ingredients and apply to clean, dry skin. Leave on for 20-30 minutes and rinse with warm water.

The Brightening Booster:

- 1/4 cup ground oatmeal
- 1 tablespoon lemon juice (diluted with water if desired)
- 1 teaspoon honey

Mix ingredients and apply to clean, dry skin, avoiding the eye area. Leave on for 10-15 minutes and rinse with cool water.

Remember, these are just starting points. Feel free to experiment and find what works best for your unique skin. And above all, enjoy the process! Embrace the self-care ritual of creating your own masks, and witness the radiant transformation that unfolds.

Three

10+ Ultimate Oatmeal Mask Recipes for Ageless Glow

Get ready to unleash your inner alchemist and whip up some magical brews for a radiant, ageless complexion! This treasure trove of 10+ oatmeal mask recipes offers something for every skin concern, from dryness and wrinkles to hyperpigmentation and sensitivity. So, grab your blender, gather your ingredients, and let's embark on a journey of DIY skincare delight!

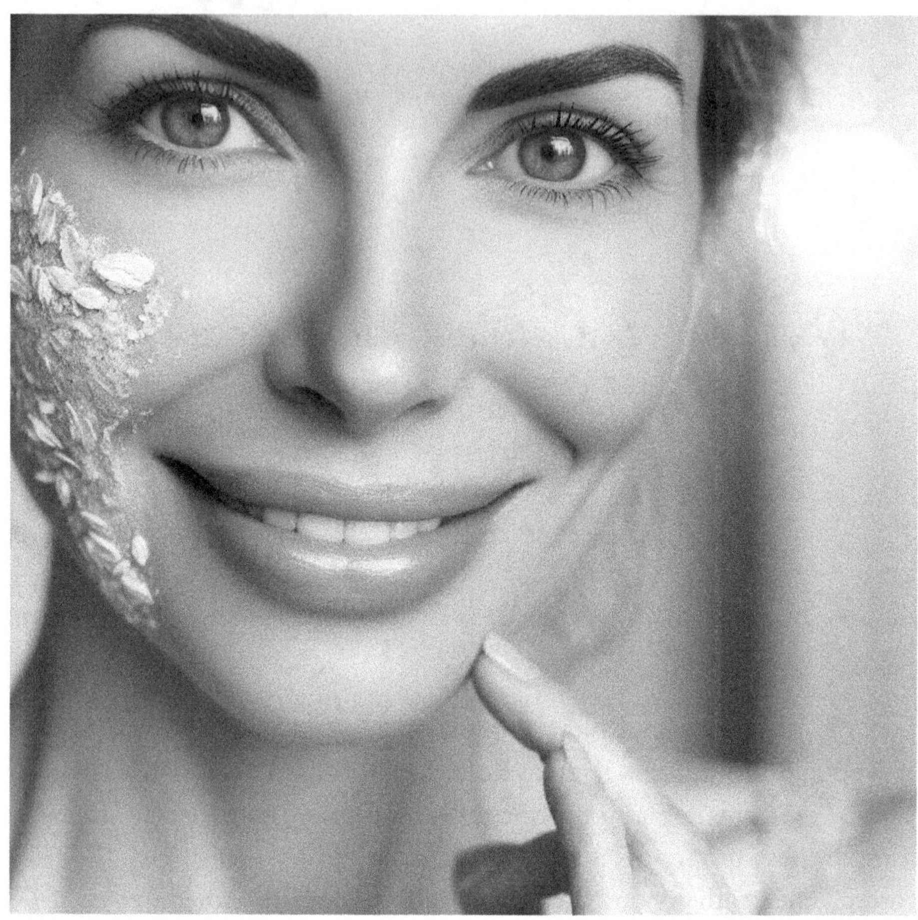

1. The Hydrating Haven: Honey-Oatmeal Mask for Deep Nourishment
Ingredients:

- 1/4 cup ground oatmeal
- 2 tablespoons plain yogurt
- 1 tablespoon honey

Benefits:

- Oatmeal: Soothes irritation, draws moisture to the skin.

- Yogurt: Provides lactic acid for gentle exfoliation, boosts hydration.
- Honey: Natural humectant, antibacterial and anti-inflammatory properties.

Instructions:

1. Blend ground oatmeal and yogurt until smooth.
2. Stir in honey and mix well.
3. Apply a generous layer to clean, dry skin, avoiding the eye area.
4. Relax for 15-20 minutes, letting the mask work its magic.
5. Rinse thoroughly with warm water and pat dry.

Tips:

- For extra hydration, add a mashed banana or avocado to the mix.
- Sensitive skin? Substitute yogurt with milk or cream for a gentler touch.
- Oily skin? Swap honey for egg white for a mattifying effect.

2. Wrinkle Rewind: Oatmeal & Retinol Mask for Firmness and Elasticity

Ingredients:

- 1/4 cup ground oatmeal
- 1/2 teaspoon retinol serum
- 1 teaspoon green tea extract

Benefits:

- Oatmeal: Soothes and calms skin, promotes collagen production.
- Retinol: Boosts collagen and elastin, reduces wrinkles and fine lines.
- Green tea extract: Rich in antioxidants, fights free radical damage.

Instructions:

1. Combine ground oatmeal and green tea extract in a bowl.
2. Add retinol serum and mix gently, avoiding contact with eyes and mouth.
3. Apply a thin layer to clean, dry skin. Leave on for 15-20 minutes, depending on your skin's sensitivity to retinol.
4. Rinse thoroughly with cool water and pat dry. Apply moisturizer with SPF as retinol increases sun sensitivity.

Tips:

- Use this mask at night, as retinol can degrade in sunlight.
- Start 1-2 times a week and gradually increase frequency based on your skin's tolerance.
- Patch test before applying to a larger area.

3. Flawless Finish: Oatmeal & Turmeric Mask for Brightening and Hyper-pigmentation

Ingredients:

- 1/4 cup ground oatmeal
- 1/2 teaspoon turmeric powder
- 1 tablespoon plain yogurt
- 1 tablespoon lemon juice (diluted with water if desired)

Benefits:

- Oatmeal: Exfoliates gently, brightens skin tone.
- Turmeric: Powerful antioxidant, reduces hyperpigmentation and evens skin tone.
- Yogurt: Lactic acid further aids in brightening and exfoliation.
- Lemon juice (optional): Natural lightening agent for stubborn spots (use with caution due to potential for irritation).

Instructions:

1. Combine ground oatmeal and turmeric in a bowl.
2. Stir in yogurt and lemon juice (if using) until you have a smooth paste.
3. Apply a thin layer to clean, dry skin, avoiding the eye area.
4. Leave on for 10-15 minutes, keeping an eye out for any tingling or discomfort.
5. Rinse thoroughly with cool water and pat dry.

Tips:

- Patch test before applying, especially if you have sensitive skin.
- Use sunscreen daily, as turmeric can increase sun sensitivity.
- Limit lemon juice usage to once or twice a week due to its potency.

4. Ageless Radiance: Oatmeal & Vitamin C Mask for Glowing Skin (300 words)

Ingredients:

- 1/4 cup ground oatmeal
- 1 teaspoon vitamin C serum
- 1 tablespoon honey
- 1/2 teaspoon rosewater

Benefits:

- Oatmeal: Soothes and hydrates, promotes healthy skin cell turnover.
- Vitamin C: Powerful antioxidant, brightens skin, boosts collagen production.
- Honey: Natural humectant, antibacterial properties.
- Rosewater: Gentle toner, calms redness and irritation.

Instructions:

1. Combine ground oatmeal and vitamin C serum in a bowl.

2. Stir in honey and rosewater until you have a smooth paste.
3. Apply a thin layer to clean, dry skin, avoiding the eye area.
4. Leave on for 15-20 minutes.
5. Rinse thoroughly with cool water and pat dry.

Tips:

- Use fresh vitamin C serum for maximum potency.
- This mask can be used 2-3 times a week for radiant skin.
- Follow with a moisturizer to lock in hydration.

5. The Youthful Lift: Oatmeal & Collagen Mask for Improved Firmness
Ingredients:

- 1/4 cup ground oatmeal
- 1 tablespoon aloe vera gel
- 1 teaspoon collagen powder
- 1/2 teaspoon avocado oil

Benefits:

- Oatmeal: Gentle exfoliation, promotes collagen production.
- Aloe vera gel: Hydrates, calms irritation, tightens pores.
- Collagen powder: Boosts collagen levels, improves skin elasticity.
- Avocado oil: Rich in fatty acids, nourishes and plumps the skin.

Instructions:

1. Combine ground oatmeal and aloe vera gel in a bowl.
2. Mix in collagen powder and avocado oil until you have a creamy paste.
3. Apply a thin layer to clean, dry skin, focusing on areas needing extra lift.
4. Leave on for 15-20 minutes.
5. Rinse thoroughly with warm water and pat dry.

Tips:

- Use marine collagen powder for optimal absorption.
- This mask can be used 2-3 times a week for firmer, plumper skin.
- Follow with a moisturizer to seal in the benefits.

6. Calm & Collected: Oatmeal & Chamomile Mask for Soothing Sensitive Skin

Ingredients:

- 1/4 cup ground oatmeal
- 1 tablespoon chamomile tea (cooled)
- 1 tablespoon plain yogurt
- 1/2 teaspoon honey

Benefits:

- Oatmeal: Soothes irritation, reduces inflammation.
- Chamomile: Anti-inflammatory properties, calms redness and itching.
- Yogurt: Gentle exfoliation, hydrates and nourishes.
- Honey: Antibacterial properties, promotes healing.

Instructions:

1. Steep chamomile tea bags in hot water for 10 minutes, then let cool.
2. Combine ground oatmeal and cooled chamomile tea in a bowl.
3. Stir in yogurt and honey until you have a smooth paste.
4. Apply a thin layer to clean, dry skin, avoiding the eye area.
5. Leave on for 15-20 minutes.
6. Rinse gently with cool water and pat dry.

Tips:

- Use this mask after sun exposure or to calm irritation from shaving.
- You can also use chilled chamomile tea bags as compresses for tired eyes.
- This mask can be used daily for sensitive skin.

7. Luxurious Spa at Home: Oatmeal & Milk Bath with Essential Oils
Ingredients:

- 1/2 cup ground oatmeal
- 1 cup dried milk powder
- 5-10 drops essential oil of your choice (lavender, rose, or chamomile recommended)

Instructions:

1. Fill your bathtub with warm water.
2. In a bowl, combine ground oatmeal and milk powder.
3. Add essential oil and mix well.
4. Tie the mixture in a cheesecloth or muslin bag and immerse it in the bathwater.
5. Soak for 15-20 minutes, allowing the oatmeal and milk to nourish and soften your skin.
6. Rinse with warm water and pat dry.

Tips:

- Use filtered water for a more luxurious experience.
- Adjust the amount of essential oil based on your preference.
- For an extra pampering touch, light candles and listen to calming music.

8. Exfoliating Delight: Oatmeal & Honey Scrub for Smoother Skin
Ingredients:

- 1/4 cup ground oatmeal

- 2 tablespoons honey
- 1 tablespoon olive oil (optional)

Instructions:

1. Combine ground oatmeal and honey in a bowl.
2. Add olive oil if desired for extra moisture.
3. Gently massage the scrub onto clean, damp skin in circular motions.
4. Focus on areas like elbows, knees, and heels.
5. Leave on for 5-10 minutes, then rinse thoroughly with warm water.
6. Follow with a moisturizer to lock in hydration.

Tips:

- Use this scrub 1-2 times a week for smoother, brighter skin.
- Be gentle around sensitive areas like the face.
- You can customize the scrub with other ingredients like lemon juice for added brightening or yogurt for additional exfoliation.

9. Targeted Treatments: Eye Masks, Lip Masks, and Spot Treatments (200 words)

The versatility of oatmeal extends beyond full-face masks. You can create targeted treatments for specific concerns:

- Eye Masks: Combine oatmeal with cucumber slices or green tea bags for puffy eyes.
- Lip Masks: Mix oatmeal with honey and avocado oil for soft, supple lips.
- Spot Treatments: Make a paste with oatmeal and honey to dab on blemishes for overnight healing.

10. Bonus Recipe: Overnight Moisture Mask for Maximum Hydration
Ingredients:

- 1/4 cup ground oatmeal
- 2 tablespoons mashed avocado
- 1 tablespoon plain yogurt
- 1 teaspoon honey

Instructions:

1. Combine all ingredients in a bowl until you have a creamy paste.
2. Apply a generous layer to clean, dry skin.
3. Leave it overnight and rinse thoroughly with warm water in the morning.

Tips:

- This mask is perfect for dry or dehydrated skin.
- You can also use it on your neck and chest for extra hydration.
- Wake up to a dewy, refreshed complexion!

Remember, this is just a starting point. Experiment, tailor these recipes to your needs, and enjoy the endless possibilities of DIY oatmeal skincare. Embrace the magic of this humble grain and unlock the ageless beauty that lies within!

Four

DIY Tips & Aftercare Secrets for Maximum Impact

Now that you're armed with a treasure trove of oatmeal mask recipes, let's unlock the secrets to maximizing their impact! By following these essential preparation, application, and aftercare tips, you'll transform your DIY sessions into luxurious rituals that nourish your skin and your soul.

Gathering Your Arsenal: Essential Tools and Kitchen Ingredients for DIY Masks

Crafting your own masks doesn't require fancy equipment. A well-stocked pantry and a few simple tools are all you need:

- Mixing bowls: Opt for glass or ceramic bowls for easy cleaning and safe mixing.
- Spoons and spatulas: Choose non-metallic utensils to avoid reactions with ingredients.
- Mesh strainer: This helps separate liquid from pulp when using fruits or vegetables.
- Applicator brush: For even application, a soft silicone brush is a gentle and hygienic choice.
- Warm towels: These come in handy for steaming and removing masks.
- Headband or clip: Keep your hair out of the way during application.

And remember, your pantry holds a wealth of natural beauty ingredients! Honey, yogurt, avocado, oatmeal (of course!), fruits, and even spices can be combined to create powerful masks for every skin concern.

Preparation is Key: Skin Cleansing and Steaming for Optimal Absorption

A clean canvas is essential for optimal mask absorption. Before diving into your DIY delight, follow these steps:

1. Cleanse your face: Remove makeup and daily grime with a gentle cleanser suitable for your skin type.
2. Exfoliate (optional): For deeper absorption, a gentle exfoliant removes dead skin cells, allowing the mask to reach deeper layers.
3. Steaming (optional): A warm steam opens pores, allowing the mask's beneficial ingredients to penetrate deeper. Drape a warm towel over your face or use a facial steamer for 5-10 minutes.

Application & Relaxation: Techniques for Effective Mask Application and Mindful Practices

Now comes the fun part! Applying your mask is a chance to indulge in self-care, so take your time and savor the process:

1. Apply with gentle fingertips: Start at your forehead and work your way down, spreading the mask evenly in a thin layer. Avoid the delicate eye area.
2. Relax and unwind: Sit back, close your eyes, and let the mask's calming properties work their magic. Light scented candles or play soothing music to enhance the experience.
3. Follow the recipe's instructions: Each mask has a specific recommended time, so set a timer to avoid over-treatment.

Gentle Removal & Aftercare: Rinsing Techniques and Skincare Routines for Long-Lasting Benefits

Once the time is up, treat your skin with the same gentle touch you used during application:

1. Rinse with lukewarm water: Avoid hot water, which can strip your skin of natural oils.
2. Pat dry with a soft towel: Don't rub, as this can irritate your skin.
3. Moisturize: Seal in the mask's benefits with a moisturizer suited to your skin type.

Remember, consistency is key. Regular DIY mask sessions will have a cumulative effect, leaving your skin glowing, hydrated, and youthful. Be patient, listen to your skin, and adjust your recipes as needed.

By embracing these tips and secrets, you'll transform your DIY oatmeal masks into powerful rituals of self-care and natural beauty. So, gather your ingredients, light some candles, and embark on a journey of ageless transformation, one spoonful of magic at a time!

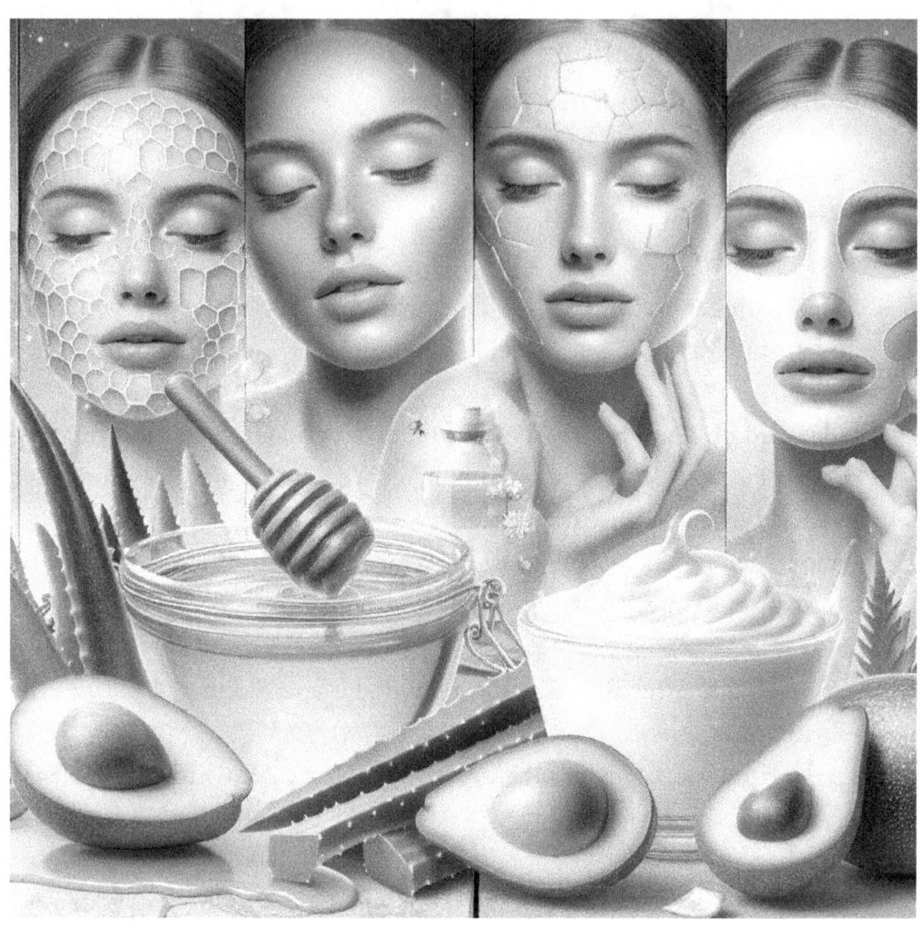

Five

Conclusion: Oatmeal – Nature's Secret Weapon for Mature Skin

As we gracefully navigate the journey of mature womanhood, our skin's needs evolve. The gentle touch of time leaves its mark, and dryness can become a frustrating foe. Yet, nestled within the humble pantry staple oatmeal lies a potent natural remedy, waiting to unveil its transformative power.

Throughout this ebook, we've explored the science behind oatmeal's magic. From its soothing colloidal properties to its antioxidant and anti-inflammatory prowess, oatmeal emerges as a champion for mature skin. Its ability to hydrate, exfoliate, and protect, all without harsh chemicals or abrasive treatments, makes it a gentle yet effective ally in your quest for a radiant complexion.

But knowledge, without action, is merely potential. So, dear reader, I invite you to embrace the power of oatmeal. Let it become an integral part of your natural skincare routine. Experiment with the DIY recipes we've shared, or seek out oatmeal-infused products crafted with care. With each application, feel the comforting embrace of nature's bounty, and witness the gradual unveiling of a healthy, luminous glow.

Embrace the Lux Within: A Call to Action

Your journey to radiant skin deserves a nurturing space, brimming with inspiration and support. At Luxskin, my natural skincare blog, you'll find a vibrant community of women like yourself, all embracing the power of nature to nourish and enhance their beauty.

Join me on this adventure, where we explore the endless possibilities of natural ingredients, celebrate self-care as a form of empowerment, and share our experiences and journeys.

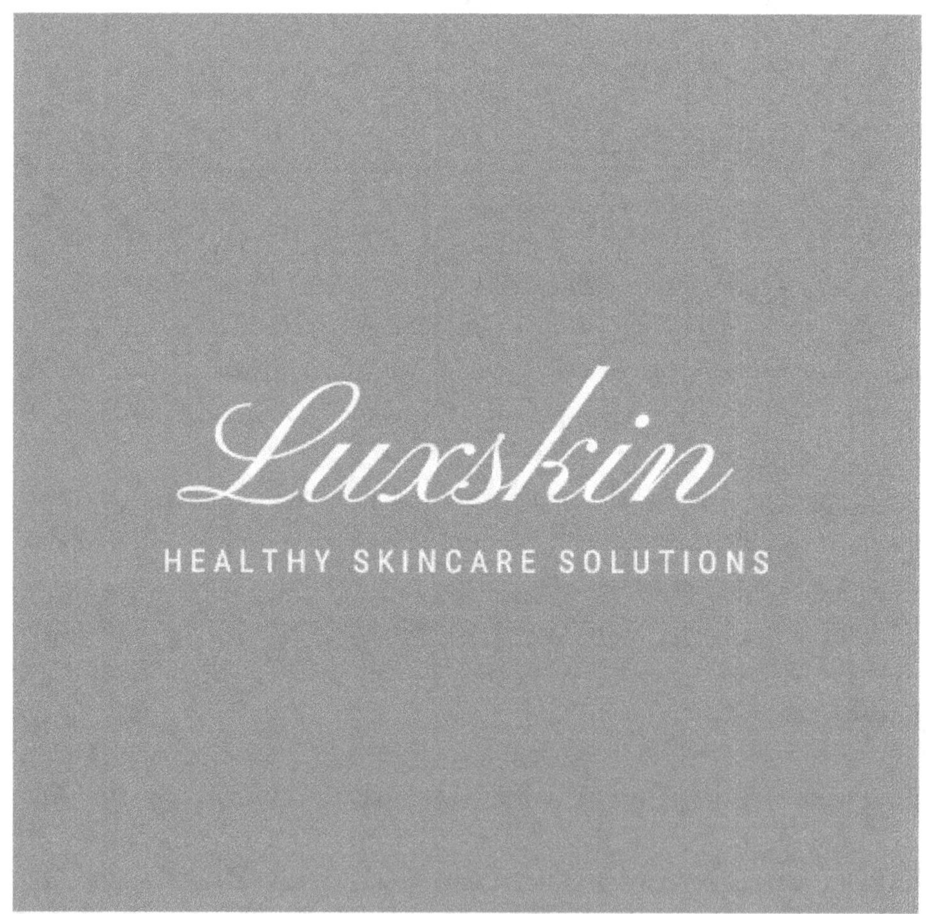

Visit Luxskin today, and let's unlock the radiant lux within, together. Share your oatmeal beauty triumphs, ask questions, and discover the endless possibilities of nature's bounty. Remember, mature skin isn't a challenge to overcome; it's a canvas waiting to be adorned with the colors of confidence, gratitude, and self-love.

With every gentle exfoliation, every nourishing mask, and every moment of self-care, you radiate a beauty that transcends time. Embrace the magic of oatmeal, nourish your skin, and let your inner lux shine through.

See you at Luxskin!

Follow me:

- Blog https://luxskin.blogspot.com
- Instagram @luxskinofficial
- Pinterest @luxskinofficial

Shop: https://luxskin/payhip.com